The 5 Biological Laws of Nature. A New Medicine
Copyright © 2018 Björn Eybl
All Rights Reserved.

7th Revised and Extended Edition
1st English Translation Edition

Translated into English by Andrew Schlademan
Cover design by Kristen Albert

ISBN-13: 978-1-948909-03-7

Library of Congress Number: 2018900188

Published by Thirty-Three & 1/ॐ Publishing

Printed and bound in the United States of America.

The author, Björn Eybl, is responsible for the content, *"Not being a physician, I am not permitted to practice medicine in Austria. Thus, I hereby point out that I have never done so. Not even with my own method. Only God, Nature and the client himself can heal."*

The content and recommendations in this book are based primarily on the scientific findings of Dr. Hamer and the author's experience with natural healing. They are meant for the reader's personal edification; they cannot, however, substitute for the diagnosis and therapy of a competent therapist. The author assumes no responsibility for recommended remedies, therapies or injury resulting there from.

The 5 Biological
Laws of Nature

A New Medicine

Björn Eybl

For therapists with heart and patients with understanding. This booklet, A New Medicine: The 5 Biological Laws of Nature, is an introduction to the desk reference book titled, The Psychic Roots of Disease: Five Biological Laws of Nature, as they were discovered and documented by Dr. Ryke Geerd Hamer, MD.

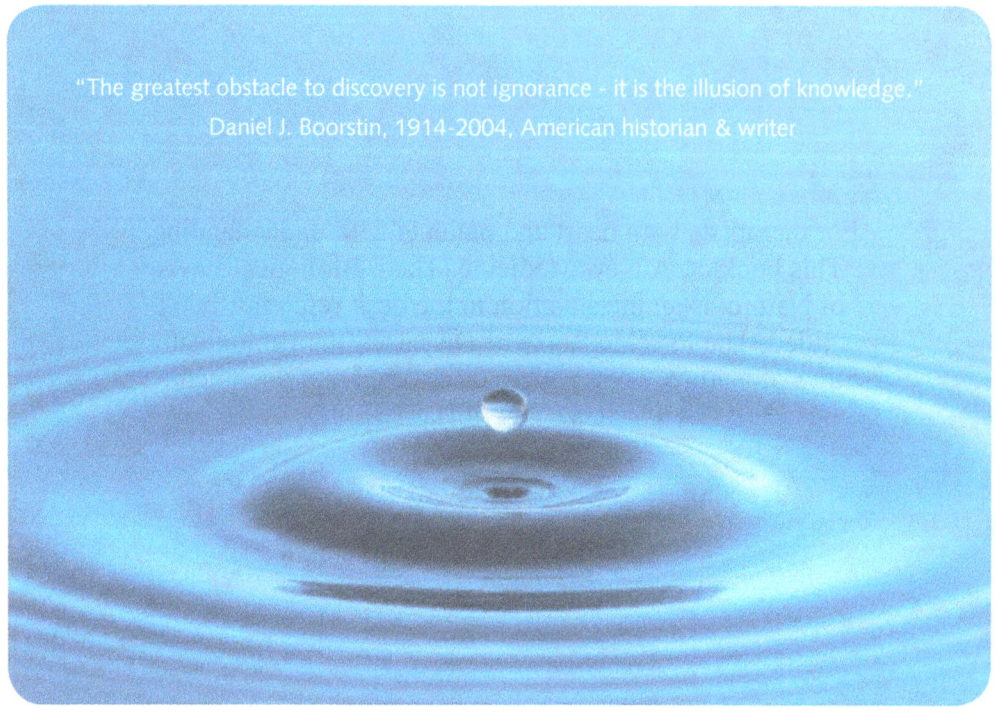

"The greatest obstacle to discovery is not ignorance - it is the illusion of knowledge."
Daniel J. Boorstin, 1914-2004, American historian & writer

Introduction

Dear reader,
Some of what you read here will seem truly incredible. That is only natural. When I explored these connections myself over 17 years ago, I couldn't believe it all either.
Fortunately, no one has to believe the New Medicine. Instead, we can all test it out ourselves - on our own bodies. For example, when you have a runny nose and come to the realization that you actually thought "That stinks!" about something beforehand. Slowly but surely, belief will become knowledge.
The five biological laws open the door to a completely new way of looking at health and illness. Conventional medicine is behind us; ahead of us lies nature in all its glory and beauty and, in close relation to it, a New Medicine which is both scientifically (bio)logical and infinitely human.
It's ironic that conventional medicine has to admit defeat in its own field when put to the test of logical reasoning.
The 5 biological laws can comprehensively explain diseases (and psychoses) and can be proven on any patient. Unlike conventional medicine it does not require any hypotheses (unproven assumptions) whatsoever.
The well-known medical journalist Peter Schmidsberger makes the point:
"If Dr. Hamer is right, then conventional medical books hold no more value than waste paper!"
In this short booklet, I would like to explain the Five Biological Laws in a simple and comprehensible way.
Even though I'll be mainly talking in relation to cancer, the five biological laws describe the cause and course of almost all diseases. These laws work, whether we are familiar with them or not and whether we believe in them or not. The laws are not only valid for humans, but for animals and, in a modified form, for plants. The

only exceptions to these laws are injuries, poisoning and diseases due to nutritional deficiencies (e.g., scurvy from vitamin C deficiency).

The Discoverer

Ryke Geerd Hamer, M.D., was born in 1935. He studied medicine, physics and theology and in 1972, he began working as specialist in internal medicine. He first worked as an intern at the University of Tübingen where he spent years working with cancer patients.

Dr. Hamer also made a name for himself through medical patents: He invented the "Hamer Scalpel," which made plastic surgery without bleeding possible. His other inventions include a special bone saw.

In 1976, his family of six (his wife was also a doctor) decided to settle in Italy where Dr. Hamer planned to open a practice for poor people. Everything was going according to plan when the family was struck by a tragic accident in 1978.

While on a boat trip, their dear son Dirk was accidentally shot by Prince Emanuel of Savoy. Drunk, the prince fired a gun and hit Dirk, asleep in another boat. After 18 operations, Dirk died in his father's arms. Three months later Dr. Hamer developed testicular cancer.

Having always been healthy up until this point, Dr Hamer began to wonder if there was a connection between the disease and the loss of his son. After his recovery he set out to answer this question and was in the perfect position to do so.

At the time, he was working as the assistant medical director in a Munich cancer clinic. He began asking the patients if they had had a shocking experience in their life before they developed the disease. Indeed, without exception they had. All 200 patients he interviewed told him of such an experience and so he reviewed their medical records in detail. When Dr. Hamer submitted his discoveries to the doctors for discussion in October of that year, he was given a choice: deny his thesis or leave the clinic. Dr. Hamer did not want to deny it and he stood his ground.

He continued his research day and night. When he left the clinic shortly after that, he was able to formulate his IRON RULE OF CANCER. From those 200 patients until today at least 40,000 cases have been examined and evaluated and not once has there been an exception.

For a long time, people had surmised that cancer could be triggered by the psyche. Finally there is now a body of scientific proof.

Until 2004, Dr. Hamer called his discovery "New Medicine." Now the title used is "German New Medicine®."

Because this name is copyrighted, I'll be talking about the New Medicine or the 5 Biological Laws in this booklet.

On July 2nd 2017, Dr. Hamer died while in exile in Norway. According to his wishes, he was buried in Erlangen, Germany. This is where he met his wife and spent the happiest years of his life.

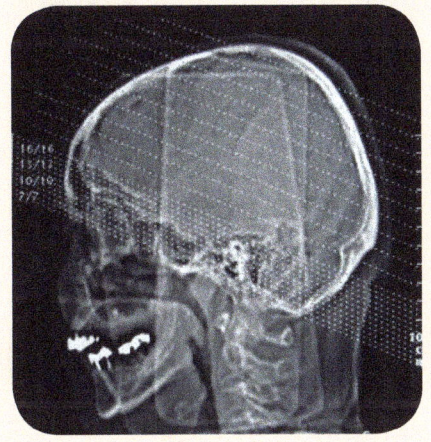

Computed tomography (CT) = Procedure of layered x-rays:
Delivers x-ray images of the brain on many parallel levels. The standard brain-CT gives about 30 photographic "cuts" through the brain.

FIRST BIOLOGICAL LAW[1]
The Conflict

1. Criteria: Every disease – from here on referred to as a Significant Biological Special Program (SBS; in the original German "Sinnvolles biologisches Sonderprogramm") – originates from a conflict shock which is very difficult, highly acute, dramatic and isolating. The shock is simultaneous on three levels: psyche, brain and organ.

2. Criteria: The conflict content, i.e. the type of feelings experienced during the shock, determines which part of the brain and in which organ an SBS manifests itself.

3. Criteria: The SBS runs its course simultaneously on the three levels: psyche, brain and organ.

A conflict shock catches an individual off guard. Given the criteria stated above, we speak of a biological conflict or a conflict from which one suffers. Small conflicts result in harmless "diseases," big conflicts result in severe "diseases."

Thinking of his son Dirk, Dr. Hamer called such a conflict shock the "Dirk Hamer Syndrome." This is a completely unexpected event which catches a person "on the wrong foot" and hits them like a crushing blow.

These do not mean everyday worries, problems and emergencies; we can adjust to or prepare for this kind of distress. A conflict shock describes the moment of surprise experienced during a dramatic event. It is when someone is personally challenged and feels completely alone in that moment. They can't or don't want to talk about the crisis (isolating).

Reason and logic are of no use to us at times like these. We experience and feel a shock. That alone counts and is enough.

At the same moment as this experience, a Significant Biological Special Program (SBS) starts and it changes our psyche, our brain and the relevant organ.

The conflict content determines which part of the brain and which organs are affected.

A practical example

A mother, holding the hand of her four-year-old daughter, is chatting to a neighbor on the sidewalk. The little girl sees a playmate on the other side of the street. Suddenly the child tears free and runs onto the street. The mother hears the screech of car tires and the next moment sees her child lying motionless on the asphalt.

The shock occurs exactly at this moment. It hits her like a crushing blow, unexpected, on the wrong foot. It's a dramatic situation and it was a surprise - a typical, biological conflict. From this moment, the young mother begins

The Hamer Focus

A serious conflict shock leaves its traces in the brain.

These spherical forms look like circular disks in brain CTs.

The arrows in the scan point out a recurring, active focus in the right side of the cerebellum. This focus correlates to the mammary glands of the left breast (mother-child-worry conflict).

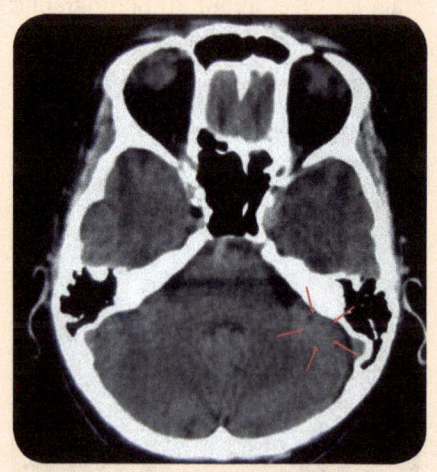

---

[1] Shortened and simplified from "KREBS und alle so. Krankheiten" by Dr. Med. Mag. Theol. Ryke Geerd Hamer, p. 28, Amici di Dirk Verlag 2004, ISBN 84-96-127-13-3

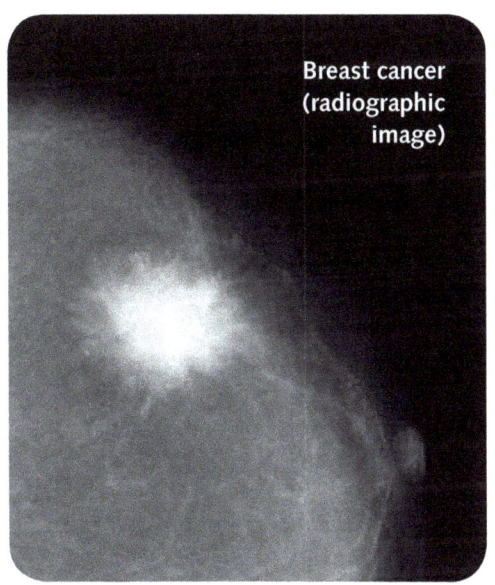

Breast cancer (radiographic image)

an SBS - in this case, a "mother-child-worry conflict."
Let's bring the example further: the child is seriously injured, the mother accompanies her daughter to the hospital. The operate on the child, her condition remains critical and the doctors don't know if the child will survive.
The woman has suffered a conflict and is now in the "conflict-active phase," also called the "cold phase."
Psyche, brain and organ are now affected:

Psyche
Continuous stress. The woman is thinking about her daughter day and night (compulsive thinking). She sleeps little and badly, has no appetite, loses weight and has cold hands.

Brain
From the instant of the conflict, we see in her cerebellum, specifically in the mammary gland center, a sharp-edged focus, called a Hamer focus (in the original German: "Hamersche Herd"), (picture below).

Organ
Metabolism is increased in the mammary gland tissue and cells divide = breast cancer.
At first glance, it might not seem to make sense, but the situation looks different when we observe it from a biological point of view.

A similar situation in the animal kingdom
One of a mother sheep's young is taken by a wolf. Immediately, she mobilizes all her reserves, runs in high gear, is under continuous stress and does everything she can to get her young back.
Through this, the mother sheep suffers from a mother-child-worry conflict, whereby her mammary gland tissue begins to increase.
In this way, more milk is made available for her young as it now requires extra nourish-

> The location of the Hamer Focus gives exact information about which organ is involved. We can also tell if the conflict is still active (sharp-edged) or if the patient is already in the repair phase (blurred edge due to water retention = edema). You could describe these Hamer foci as the fingerprints of the psyche.
> They are the living proof that above the brain, the psyche controls all organs.
> In the picture, you can see two sharp-edged Hamer foci (relays for the larynx and bronchi), which means that the conflicts are still active, i.e., not yet resolved.

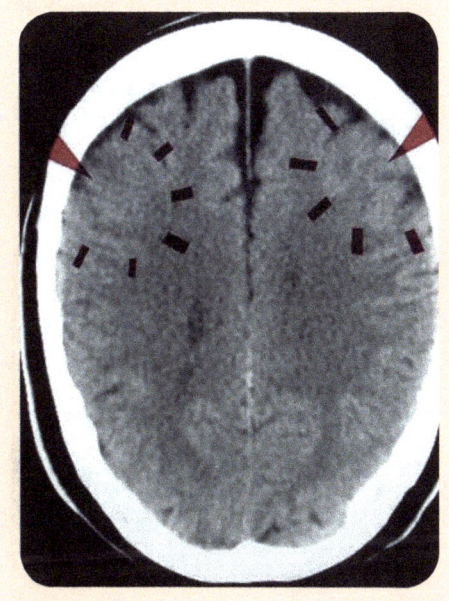

ment for a quick recovery.
This is the precise biological meaning: a gift of nature, which still makes complete sense among peoples living with little or no contact with civilization - a quick recovery is made possible for an injured infant.

Now back to our case example
Her child is still in the hospital. The mother is still under constant stress. As long as the mother-child-worry conflict continues, the breast cancer grows.
Weeks later the doctor reports:
"Your daughter has made it. She won't suffer from any lasting damage."
Without a doubt, the best news the mother could imagine = conflict resolution.
From this exact moment the repair phase begins:
She is happy about life again. Even though she would like to sleep day and night, she's fatigued and has a headache (from the swelling in the brain, in this case the cerebellum = repair of the Hamer focus).
Her appetite returns and her hands are hot. But most importantly: the recently increased mammary gland tissue begins decreases again.
If you were to examine the breast in this phase, you would be more likely to assume the opposite. The breast is now hot and swollen. The lump is now larger than before. However, these are the welcome signs of healing, because tuberculosis bacteria are now at work, removing the excess mammary gland tissue - more about that later.
The organ in which a Significant Biological Special Program (SBS) starts is determined by the kind of experience during the conflict shock.

Another example:
A woman catches her husband in bed with another woman. She can experience this in different ways:
• E.g., as a "female territorial-loss conflict": "Why is he having sex with her and not me?" - affected organ: cervix
• or as a "self-esteem conflict" ("I can't compete with this young woman") - affected organ: cervix musculature
• or a "fear-revulsion conflict" (if, for example, it's a prostitute), when it appears organically as hypoglycemia (pancreas)
• or a "territorial-marking conflict" ("That is my husband and he belongs to my territory") UTI - bladder infection (cystitis) in the repair phase
• or she doesn't love her husband anymore and has a boyfriend herself = no conflict, no SBS. Every one of these SBSs is "tailor-made" and fulfills a very specific biological purpose.

"Brain Tumor"
A Hamer focus after the conflict was resolved: the sharp-edged rings are no longer visible. The blurred edge is made up of residual, radiopaque contrast medium. Conventional medicine calls this stage of healing a "malignant brain tumor."
In the experience of New Medicine, these formations are harmless.
In established medicine, a lot of patients die from fear, panic and from "therapy" (chemo and radioactive irradiation).

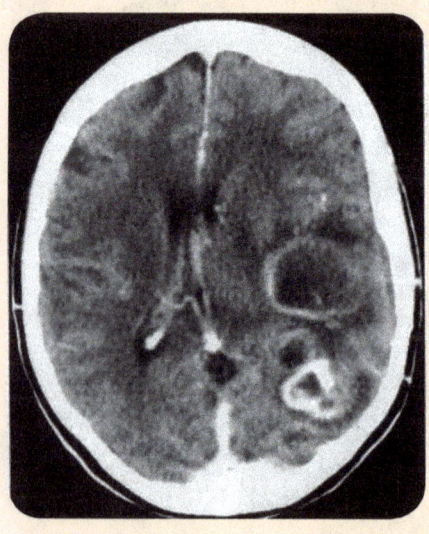

SECOND BIOLOGICAL LAW[2]
The Two-Phased Process

In conventional medicine, we know of the autonomic nervous system with its two opposing branches, the active nerve (sympathicotonia) and the calm nerve (parasympathicotonia/vagotonia).

The **sympathicotonic** system controls the bodily functions during waking hours (work, sports, stress).

The **vagotonic** system takes over during rest, relaxation and recuperation.

In the normal day and night rhythm, the two parts swap back and forth evenly, like the pendulum of a clock (as in the left column of the diagram below).

Dr. Hamer has, however, discovered that after a conflict shock, the body automatically "switches over" into continuous stress. Every one of us can observe this in ourselves: an accident happens – extreme distress (biological conflict): instantly we get cold hands, lose our appetite, heartbeat and breathing speed up and our thoughts are occupied by just one thing. We are now in the "cold phase," in continuous stress, called **"conflict-active."** The sympathicotonic system reigns even at night now: we sleep badly or not at all (see second column of diagram).

Let's recall the mother with the "concern-conflict" for her child. She doesn't know if her child will survive the accident. She has cold hands, little appetite, she barely sleeps.

For weeks, the pendulum stays in extreme sympathicotonia. Then, the resolving news: "Your child will make a full recovery!"

After this good news, the pendulum swings equally hard to the other side. The woman falls into strong vagotonia; the second phase, the **repair phase**, has begun.

This includes: hot hands, healthy appetite, the

---

[2] Shortened and simplified from "KREBS und alle so. Krankheiten" by Dr. Med. Mag. Theol. Ryke Geerd Hamer, p. 44, Amici di Dirk Verlag 2004, ISBN 84-96-127-13-3

The course of an illness if the conflict is resolved – our most important graph*

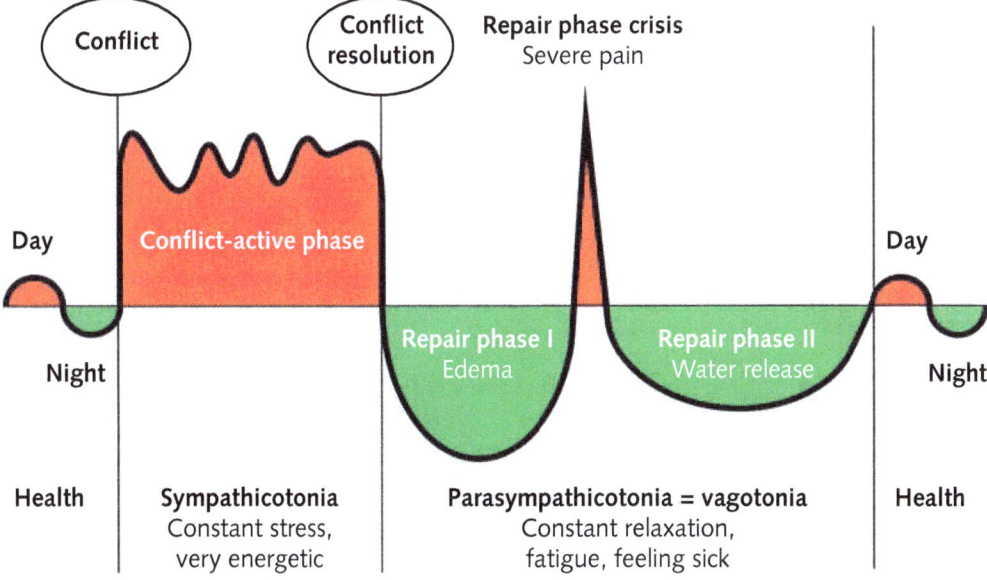

* Cf. "Dr. Hamer, German New Medicine®–Brief Information " pp. 14, 15

need to sleep, fever, headache, and of course, the sore, swollen breast.

This repair phase, also called the "warm phase" lasts, at most, as long as the conflict-active phase.

The repair phase is interrupted approximately half way through by the **repair phase crisis** (see column 3 of diagram).

This time is the most critical during the whole cycle. The most well known healing crises are epileptic seizures and heart attacks. Often, during these "cold days," we experience the conflict again, both emotionally and physically, as if in an instant replay.

Left or Right Handed? The clap test

Handedness is very important for us. It is fixed in our brains (even before birth) and remains the same for life.

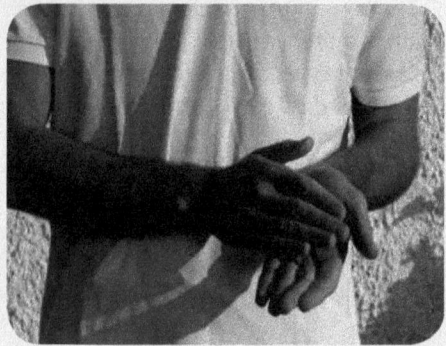

Right hand above: biological right-hander

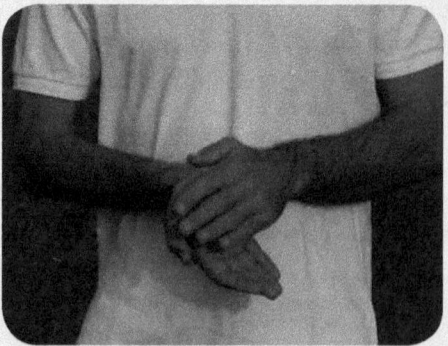

Left hand above: biological left-hander

Clap your hands and observe which hand leads. This is the one that lies on top or actively claps. It's possible you are left-handed, even if you thought that you were right-handed until now, because many people were retrained as children.

Ascertaining someone's handedness is one of the most important aspects of New Medicine because a simple rule follows from this knowledge:

The left side of the body is the mother/child side (own mother, own children, or people and animals about whom you feel this way).

The right side of the body is the partner side (father, siblings, business or life partners, colleagues, friends, enemies, relatives). With left-handed people, regardless of gender, it is the exact opposite.

For instance, if the left knee is giving a right-handed person problems, then it has to do with their mother or children. (Knees have to do with "self-esteem conflict of being non-athletic/mobile" - in this case, in relation to their mother or children.)

A painful left shoulder in a left-handed person points to an overwhelming "self-esteem conflict in relation to a partner" (someone other than mother or children). For example, guilty feelings: "What a terrible partner I am!"

Our case example:

If the woman whose child was in the accident, is a right-hander, then we already know which breast is affected: the left mother/child breast.

Have a look sometime at how a right-hander carries their child: the child's face usually lies on their left breast. That is why the SBS starts in the left breast.

During this crisis, the rudder is turned back in the direction of a normal condition again. The edemas in the brain and organ are squeezed out (water release). This is why the healing crisis is followed by the so-called "pee-pee phase."

Country doctors of old knew this critical phase well. Back then they used to say, "If he survives the next few days, then he's over the worst!"

Unfortunately our modern doctors know barely anything about this anymore.

This is why no one can explain, for example, why heart attacks almost always occur during states of relaxation and calm (at the beginning, during and at the end of the weekend). If the "clogged coronary vessels" were to blame, as conventional medicine claims, then they should occur during physical exertion (work, sport).

In fact, a heart attack is the healing crisis of a "territorial-loss conflict" (unwanted retirement, being fired, their partner leaves them, etc.), which can only end fatally if the conflict has been active for more than nine months.

The interesting thing about the second biological law is the fact that most of the symptoms of "disease" only arise in the second phase and are actually symptoms of "healing"(colds, coughs, urinary tract infections, neurodermatitis, etc.) and no longer need therapy.

Only a fool would try to "cure" something that is already in the process of healing.

If a person can't resolve a conflict at all, it leads to emaciation and eventually complete wasting. The organism becomes weaker and weaker until it eventually dies.

If the conflict can't be resolved, it's better if we can at least manage within the framework of the conflict. This is to say, even though the conflict is still active, we manage to live with it (the „downwardly transformed" conflict).

THE THIRD BIOLOGICAL LAW[3]

The Ontogenetic System of "Diseases" or Germ Layer Order

Dr. Hamer observed the following: on the one hand, there are types of cancer in which tumors grow during the conflict-active phase and disappear again during the repair phase.

On the other hand, there are cancers in which the opposite is the case; cells are destroyed during the conflict-active phase and this is repaired with the development of new tissue during the repair phase. So, these are formations or tumors that only appear in the repair phase.

How is this supposed to make sense?

Dr Hamer solved this puzzle with the help of embryology and the knowledge of the meaning of the three embryonic germ layers:

In conventional medicine, we recognize the inner (endoderm), middle (mesoderm) and outer (ectoderm) germ layers. For example, the digestive tract is formed in the endoderm, the motor skills in the mesoderm and sensory organs and skin in the ectoderm.

However, Dr. Hamer also discovered that each one of these "tissue types" is controlled by a specific part of the brain and reacts to very specific conflicts with either **cell growth** or **cell degradation**.

He discovered that the "inner germ layer organs," which are controlled by the brain stem, grow cells in the stress phase and destroy cells in the repair phase, the "middle layer" organs, which are controlled by the cerebellum, act in the same way.

The organs of the middle and outer germ layers that are controlled by the cerebrum, the cerebral white matter and the cerebral cortex behave in the completely opposite way. In the conflict phase, cells are degraded and then are restored in the repair phase.

Some organs have parts of more than one germ layer, which complicates things some-

---

[3] Shortened and simplified from "KREBS und alle so. Krankheiten" by Dr. Med. Mag. Theol. Ryke Geerd Hamer, p. 67, Amici di Dirk Verlag 2004, ISBN 84-96-127-13-3

The order of the embryonic germ layers

Endoderm or inner germ layer (brain stem)	Mesoderm „Old-Mesoderm" (cerebellum)	Mesoderm „New-Mesoderm" (cerebral white matter)	Epidermis or outer germ layer (cerebral cortex)
Digestive organs, kidney manifolds, alveoli, uterine lining, prostate gland, smooth muscular system and more	Inner and outer skin: dermis, heart sac, peritoneum, pulmonary pleura, mammary glands and more	Supporting and connective tissue: bones, cartilage, tendons, sinews, nourishment of the striped muscles, blood vessels, ovaries and more	Sensory organs, epidermis, cardiac arteries and veins, disk epithelium, laryngeal and bronchial mucous membrane, tooth enamel and more
Want/don't want conflicts – not getting or being able to get rid of a thing or what you do/don't deserve	Injuries to integrity, having one's name besmirched, attack, concern, argument or nest conflict	Self-esteem conflicts, lack of self-trust, doubt about whether one is good enough	Social conflicts, separation conflicts, territorial-loss conflicts, disgust or rejection conflicts and more
Conflict-active Increased functioning, cell augmentation/ adeno-ca (tissue growth)	**Conflict-active** Increased functioning, cell augmentation/ compact-ca (tissue growth)	**Conflict-active** Loss of function, cell degradation/ necrosis-ca (tissue degradation)	**Conflict-active** Loss of function, cell degradation/ epithelial ulcerous-ca (tissue degradation)
Repair phase Normalization of functioning, cell degradation	**Repair phase** Normalization of functioning, cell degradation	**Repair phase** Increased functioning, cell growth	**Repair phase** Increased functioning, cell growth

what, but let's look at it all in terms of our breast-cancer case example:
During the conflict-active phase the mother developed extra mammary gland cells, which are controlled by the cerebellum. In the repair phase, the surplus tissue will be removed again under orders from the cerebellum.
However, the breasts also consist of ectodermal tissue, namely the milk ducts, which lead the milk out to the nipple.
The milk ducts represent entirely different conflict content, for example, "my child or partner was torn from my breast." We call this a "separation conflict." These separation conflicts cause a Hamer focus to develop in the cerebral cortex ... (continued on page 15). If the mother had experienced the accident in this way, which would have also been a very plausible reaction, her milk ducts would have reacted with cell degeneration during the conflict-active phase.
The missing cell layers would have been rebuilt during the repair phase – this time under the orders of the cerebral cortex.
Admittedly, the interconnectedness between conflict perception, handedness and the different germ layers is probably quite confusing at first, but you don't have to understand everything all at once. For a deeper understanding, you can read "The Psychic Roots of Disease" by Björn Eybl, the "Scientific Chart of Germanic New Medicine®" by Dr. Hamer and also access the many Internet websites on the subject. The main thing is: We now understand that all processes of the body follow a specific system. We know which areas of the brain and organs are affected by which conflicts and we know exactly what happens there.
We know, for instance, that a "stink conflict" ("I can't stand that!") causes a Hamer focus to form in the cerebral cortex and also cell degeneration in the nasal mucous membrane. These cells are regenerated in the repair phase – commonly called a head cold.
An "intellectual self-esteem conflict" ("I'm way too stupid for this work!") produces a Hamer focus in the cerebral white matter and cell degeneration in the neck (cervical) area of the spine. During the repair phase, bone substance is restored (= neck-ache).

Varying behaviors of the embryonic germ layers using an example from the breast

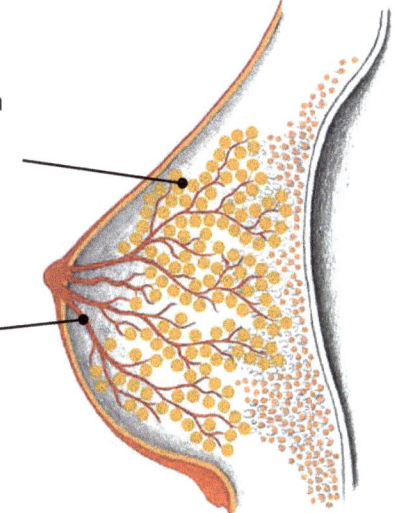

The mammary glands
belong to the middle germ layer or mesoderm
(cerebellum = old-mesoderm)
> cell generation in the conflict-active phase
> cell degradation in the repair phase
Conflict: concern, dispute or nest conflict

The milk ducts (lactiferous ducts)
belong to the outer germ layer or ectoderm
(cerebral cortex)
> cell destruction in the conflict-active phase
> cell generation in the repair phase
Conflict: separation conflict

Image according to the graphic of Dr. Hamer, Wissenschaftliche Tabelle der Neuen Medizin, cover p. 3, above left, Amici di Dirk Verlag.

THE FOURTH BIOLOGICAL LAW[4]
The Ontogenetic System of Microbes

In conventional medicine, microbes are divided into "good" (intestinal, mouth and vaginal flora) and "bad" (e.g., tubercle bacillus/*Mycobacterium tuberculosis*).

People still think that the "bad" ones are to blame for many illnesses. People call these illnesses "infectious diseases." This serious mistake happened because people did in fact find bacteria or fungi in the area of these diseases. Let's make a comparison with someone analyzing the reasons behind building fires:

"I've evaluated all of the major fires of the last decade. The result is clear. Without exception the fire department was present at every fire. Thus, these personnel and their vehicles are clearly the cause of the fires."

Of course that's nonsense. As everyone knows, fire departments don't cause fires, but they put them out. It's the exact same with fungi, bacteria and viruses. They do not cause the disease, but participate in the recovery.

Microbes have been our loyal companions for millions of years. We live in perfect symbiosis with them. Our brains and bodies count on them. The brain gives them the order to go into action for very specific operations. Our little micro-surgeons build tissue or destroy it – and only in the repair phase:

Fungi and mycobacteria, our oldest companions, take their orders from the brain stem and clear away excess tissue in the endodermal or-

---

[4] Shortened and simplified from "KREBS und alle so. Krankheiten" by Dr. Med. Mag. Theol. Ryke Geerd Hamer, p. 74, Amici di Dirk Verlag 2004, ISBN 84-96-127-13-3

The steering of microbes by the parts of the brain

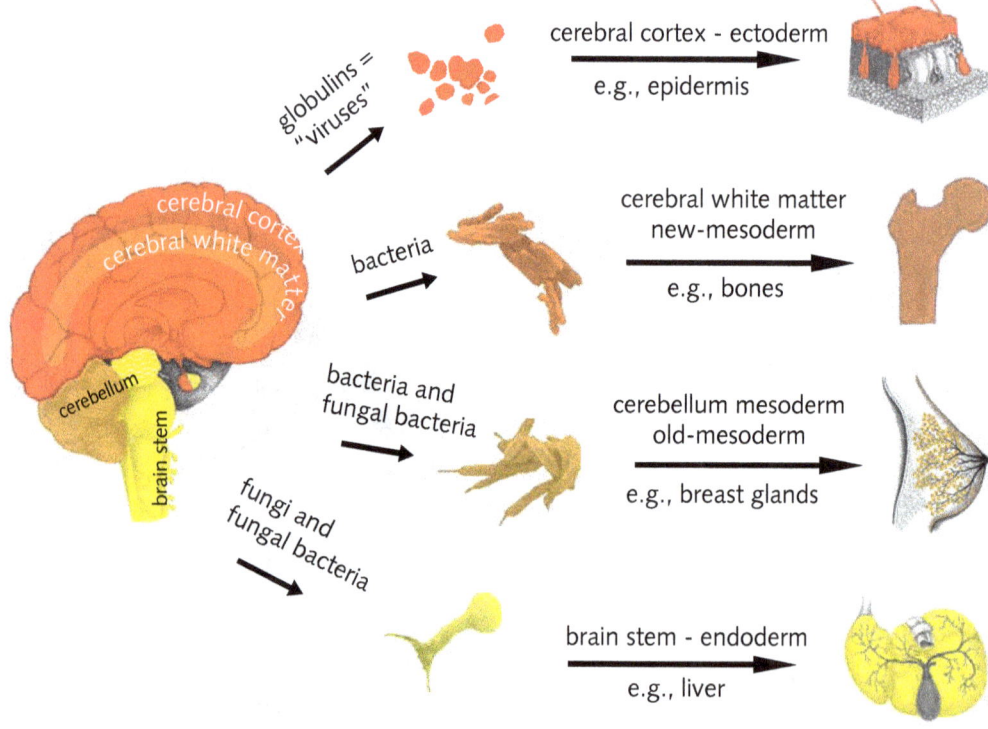

gans (e.g. candida fungus in the intestines, thrush in the mouth). Night sweats are a sure sign that they are in action.

There are different types of bacteria and each one works in a specific location e.g., gonococci bacteria appears in the urogenital system and corynebacteria in the throat.

Some bacterias are controlled by the cerebellum and destroy tissue (e.g. breast tumors), others are controlled by the cerebral cortex and build up tissue (e.g. cartilage, bones).

It's possible (it's not fully researched yet) that the cerebrum, the youngest part of our brains, works with tiny protein bonds (so-called viruses) to complete missing tissue in the repair phase (e.g. bronchi, skin).

Microbes are important members of nature's control system. We should celebrate them instead of fighting them. (Inside us, they outnumber our own body's cells by 4:3)! From the point of view of the Five Biological Laws, immunizations are not only pointless (because they are ineffective) but also extremely damaging because of the toxic additives (phenol, formaldehyde, mercury, aluminum compounds, nanoparticles and others).

If, for example, mycobacteria is missing because it's been killed it off through the use of antibiotics, then excess tissue cannot be degraded.

The body has to help in a different way: it encapsulates the tumor in connective tissue (fibrosis) and cuts it off from the metabolism.

Thus, in an x-ray of a breast, we find old calcified knots which were once milk-producing cells of an SBS.

What nature didn't plan for was modern travel. We can now be in distant countries within hours and find ourselves circulating within whole worlds of microbes that are unfamiliar to our bodies. This can lead to problems, but we see that birds have adapted rather well.

FIFTH BIOLOGICAL LAW[5]

The Biological Reason for "Diseases"

Significant Biological Special Program (SBS) – the name already points to it: every "disease" has a specific meaning. To understand the meaning of "diseases," in and of themselves, is surely the most valuable gift of the New Medicine, comparable with the feeling of happiness a blind person must have when they can suddenly see again.

Before, when people used to look for the meaning behind diseases, they would think they had something to do with fate or God's punishment. Conventional medicine didn't spend much time questioning why. Contemporary medicine assumes that all humans are just sacks full of chemical elements, coincidental products of chance and therefore prone to error.

It's only thanks to the Five Biological Laws that we can finally recognize that mother nature has always meant well for all and keeps everything in good order.

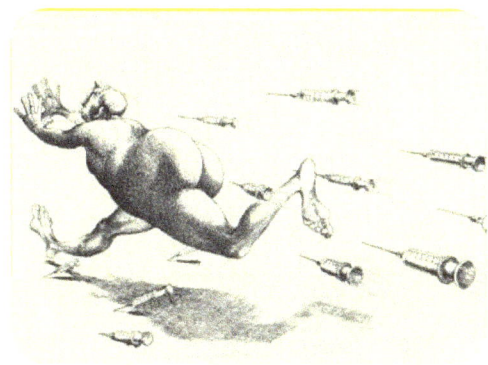

These SBSs are age-old and have been proven over millions of years. They only start when an organism is confronted with an exceptional situation and is caught off guard.

"Benign" or "malignant"?

Whether a tumor (growth) is "benign" or "malignant" (from Latin = good/evil) depends on various criteria according to conventional

---

5 Shortened and simplified from "KREBS und alle so. Krankheiten" by Dr. Med. Mag. Theol. Ryke Geerd Hamer, p. 78, Amici di Dirk Verlag 2004, ISBN 84-96-127-13-3

medicine. Apart from size, appearance and the growth behavior of the tumor, the main deciding factor is the microscopic findings (biopsy): If upon microscopic analysis, many enlarged cells are found and these have enlarged nuclei, then the diagnosis is "malignant" (see pictures below).

To explain: tissue growth always functions the same way inside the body:

First, the cell swells. The nucleus and other cell components multiply. Shortly before dividing, the cell is almost double the size as it was before. Now, it cuts into itself and divides. We end up with two cells instead of one.

The "offspring" is noticeable by its large cells in comparison to the rest of the mass.

Instead of "malignant," it would be correct to speak of "growing tissue." The conventional medical boundary between "malignant" and "benign" is anything but clear.

Histologists often disagree with each other - namely when the tissue growth has just begun or has almost come to a standstill.

Until now, we didn't know why tissue suddenly began growing. We thought it was an "error of nature" and called it "malignant." Through the Five Biological Laws, we now know that tissue doesn't just begin growing for no reason. Instead, it is to do with an SBS, which is controlled by the brain.

According to this logic, when embryonic tissue or that of a healing wound is examined under a microscope, it would have to categorized as "malignant" tissue growth.

Enlarged cells and enlarged nuclei indicate that tissue growth is active.

The connective tissue of a healing, broken bone does not differ from bone cancer tissue. It is comparable to the repair phase of a self-esteem conflict involving cell growth.

Another example

During pregnancy, women's breasts enlarge as the mammary gland cells increase. Without knowledge of the pregnancy, a histological examination would return a result of "malignant breast cancer."

It's the same with a woman who is experiencing an active "worry conflict" (malignant breast cancer). In this case, the milk ducts are also growing. If the "worry conflict" is resolved, the

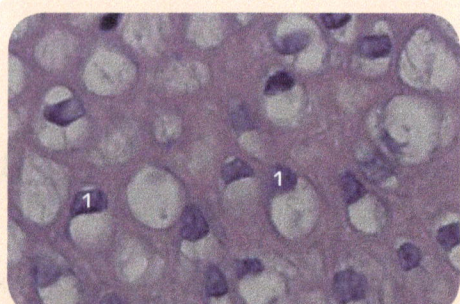

Both images show cervical smear tests of two women (400x magnification).
On the first image, we see cells of almost the same size with faint, small, normal-sized cell nuclei (1).
Only a few are in division = not-growing tissue. Finding of conventional medicine: "benign and regular, respectively."
(Source of both images: pathology from a clinic).

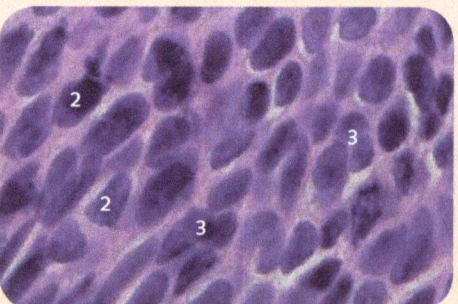

On this image we see cells with highly enlarged cell nuclei (2).
The dark coloration of the compound shows an increased cell metabolism.
Some cells are proliferating (3).
Altogether a clear indication for growing tissue. Finding of conventional medicine: "malignant." Finding of the New Medicine: repair phase of a female territorial-loss conflict.

cell division stops. Examined during this phase, the diagnosis is: "benign breast cancer." Now people think, "Phew! That was lucky!"

You see, this classification into "benign" and "malignant" is a relic from the Middle Ages and has as little to do with science as "the battle between good and evil." Back then, people were required to believe in God and Satan, heaven and hell. Today, people are told the fairy-tale of "benign cancer" and "malignant cancer," "metastasis" and "dangerous viruses." The intention is the same today as it was then: to keep people in a state of fear and dependence, in order to take the money from their pockets.

Back then, they made people dependent on the state-sanctioned church. Today, people dependent on the state-sanctioned, pharmaceutical-medical industry.

What is the meaning of increased mammary gland tissue (= breast cancer)?

More mammary gland tissue produces more breast milk. This extra milk is available to the child. Mother nature wants the child to recover quickly. This is why more nourishment is made ready. As long as the conflict continues, the tumor continues to grow. The child can drink from the "full cup" and quickly catch up with any setbacks caused by the accident.

This age-old SBS still completely fulfills its purpose among primitive peoples. As necessary, the breast was even given to other family members when they were ill. Unimaginable today, but nature isn't bothered by how "modern" (= removed from nature) our lives are today.

The SBS - real or figurative meaning? A case of bowel cancer

As far as we're concerned, evolution has been taking place forever. While species have competed with each other to eat, the human species has also competed among itself to eat and reproduce. All living things experience the conflicts that come along with survival.

The behaviors and trappings of civilization, so important to us, were never foreseen by Mother Nature. Our modern emotions are real, but they correspond to much deeper-seated SBSs.

For example, a man trusts his business partner with a large sum of money. Suddenly, he realizes he's been had! Like a "chunk/morsel" of food stuck inside him, he "can't digest" the betrayal. Suffering an "indigestible-anger" or "being-outsmarted" conflict, his psyche interprets his conflict about money as a chunk/morsel conflict and his large intestine starts producing cells immediately **to help absorb and utilize the "morsel"** - as long as the conflict exists. This may seems absurd, but for a wolf with a bone stuck in his gut, it's a life-saver.

The meaning of testicular cancer?

Cell growth in the gonads starts when a man has gone through a "loss conflict," because, e.g., his son or wife dies, his daughter moves away forever, his beloved cat gets run over etc. In the conflict-active phase, cells are destroyed to initiate, so to speak, the repair phase in which new testicular cells are produced. In fact, there are now more than before.

That's exactly the point: the now enlarged testicles produce more testosterone (male sexual hormone) and more sperm. The testosterone flood jump-starts the man sexually and the extra sperm takes care of **replacing the loss** quickly.

The reason one's psyche makes no differentiation between the loss of a son and that of a cat is something for future study. However, when one is so fond of a pet that they interpret its loss as a threat to survival, this age-old program starts running, allowing for quick reproduction.

The female equivalent is ovarian cancer. Here, once the "loss conflict," is resolved, it results in an increase in ovarian activity, providing a flood of estrogen.

Thus, the woman is very receptive to sex, likelier to conceive and is even more attractive to males! Ideal reproductive conditions. Here, nature wants to "engender" a quick replacement.

Dermatitis signals a survived "separation conflict." The biological meaning of this SBS lies in the conflict-active phase, which most people don't notice because the symptoms are barely apparent.

When, for example, we are really suffering because we no longer have skin contact with a loved one, the skin begins to go numb and to flake off at exactly the spot where we crave their touch. Cell degradation is underway.

At the same time, our short term memory is affected; the purpose of the numbness is to **block out or "forget" the touch we miss**.

We pay the price of this natural help during the repair phase: the skin regenerates under redness, swelling and an itchy rash. This process is called neurodermatitis.

If the dermatitis keeps coming back, it's because the separation conflict keeps recurring. However, it's also possible that we are repeatedly reminded of it by the circumstances surrounding the conflict (smells, people, food, music, etc.). These so-called triggers start the SBS anew every time (= allergy).

Pain in physical movement serves the purpose of getting a creature to stay still. Just as a car has to stop to be repaired, bones, cartilage, tendons and muscles can only heal in a state of relaxation.

In the case of bones, active metabolic processes take place under the periosteum (inflammation). When the tissue has regenerated, the pain disappears. After the SBS, the bone is in fact even **stronger than before** ("luxury group").

Bronchial cancer

Here, the meaning also lies in the conflict-active phase. If a living creature suffers a "territorial-fear conflict" (e.g. a successful manager is afraid that a younger, cleverer colleague could take his place or a stepmother moves into a household and keeps interfering in her stepdaughter's business), a meaningful biological program starts with cell degradation in the bronchial mucous membrane.

This enlarges the opening to the bronchi which results in **increased breathing ability**.

That is exactly the purpose, because only with extremely strenuous effort can a rival can be thrown out of the territory.

We usually pay the price of this short term increase in performance in the form of bronchitis or bronchial cancer during the repair phase = infection and swelling during the reconstruction of the mucous membrane.

"Metastases"

One of the many assumptions of conventional medicine that there are "metastases." They imagine that cancer cells wander off and settle somewhere in another organ.

The fact remains: not one cancer cell has ever been found or proven to be present in one drop of arterial blood.

If this were the case, conventional medicine would obviously want to test the blood from blood donors for cancer cells because of the danger of transfer – this, however, is not done. Ask your doctor sometime why this is! You'll get the most incredible answers.

What then are "metastases," if they don't exist?

These so-called "daughter cells" are newly developed cancers from the shock of the conventional medical death diagnoses and prognoses like:

"Sorry, we've discovered a malignant breast cancer."

When you hear something like this and are unfamiliar with the Five Biological Laws, it hits you like a blow from a sledgehammer. Most people can hardly imagine anything worse.

If the patient feels, for instance, the fear of death in this moment, a new SBS begins immediately.

The "death-fright conflict" leads to cell growth in the alveoli.

Within weeks they will find so-called coin lesions in the lungs (= lung cancer). With this SBS, the body tries to help itself by producing extra alveoli. It connects the fear of death with not getting enough air to breathe.

At the same time, the woman may experience a "self-esteem conflict":

"Without a breast, I no longer have any value as a woman!" In this case, a SBS starts on the thoracic spine or the ribs. This will be called bone cancer by conventional medicine.

This explains why we hardly ever find metastases ("secondary cancer" would be correct) in animals.

Thankfully, a dog doesn't understand when the vet says to his master: "Your dog has cancer." Usually, Rex just wags his tail and is happy the examination is over. That's why he doesn't experience a new conflict or a second cancer.

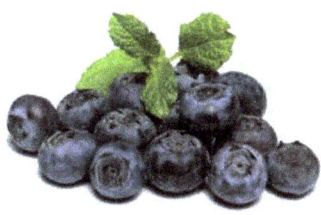

Therapy

Therapy in New Medicine, first of all, consists of explaining the biological connections to the patient. The most important thing for the patient is to understand what is happening in the body. Fear and panic are the biggest pitfalls on the road to healing.

People can put up with even intense pain when they realize that it is a part of the repair phase, that it will pass and that it has a purpose. Any actions that strengthen the morale and self-healing powers of the body are useful. Since most symptoms first arise during the repair phase, one "therapy" session is usually enough. Medications and operations are not dismissed out of principle. Of course, modern trauma medicine can work wonders after accidents. For diseases, surgical intervention is useful for clearing an intestinal blockage or when a tumor grows too large and affects other organs (this should be common sense). Operations, e.g., for cataracts are sensible, as well as artificial hip implants when the conflict resolution doesn't work and all other possibilities have been exhausted.

Additionally, the whole spectrum of natural medicine is "allowed" to be used. "God's pharmacy" (e.g. herbs, water) is available to everyone for a reason.

Dr. Hamer's thoughts on chemotherapy: "To sell it as therapy is perhaps the greatest deceit in medicine to this day. Whoever thought up chemo-torture as a therapy deserves to have a monument erected to them in hell."

Why are more and more people dying of cancer?

• Medical check-ups: I quote Dr. Roithinger, the late Austrian physician:

"Medical check-ups are the last possibility for recruiting a healthy person into the health care system." In this context, he also spoke of them as a "dragnet."

Example: breast cancer check-ups. Almost every woman will experience at least one small lump in her breast during the course of her lifetime. Earlier, they were simply ignored and nobody made a big deal about them. Today, women are prodded, x-rayed and, as necessary, biopsies are performed. > Thus, many women go from being healthy to being cancer patients from one day to the next. In this process, they experience the shock of the diagnosis and submit themselves, full of hopes and fears, to conventional medicine's sometimes deadly therapies.

• Every trifle is immediately examined – if you search for it, you'll find it – an exact diagnosis must be produced. Example: Earlier, the family doctor would send a patient with a headache, double-vision and dizziness to their bed for a week. Today this is immediately examined in all detail. This means they will be sent to a radiologist for a CT scan and they will look for a cause. In doing so, the diagnosis often comes back as a "brain tumor" (mortality rate: approximately 98%).

• Our life is becoming ever more "removed from nature" and dis-eased: constant stress in normal "everyday life," stress and shocks through artificial stimulus (smart phones, TV news and "entertainment"), poisoning by industrial-chemical nutrition, pesticides, vaccinations, chemtrails, electro-smog (e.g., cell phones, Wi-Fi and other electromagnetic interference), also poisons in our water (hormones, residual pharmaceuticals, fluoride, chlorine), medications (e.g. antibiotics = mini-chemotherapy), in cosmetics and much, much more.

Does everyone survive with the New Medicine?

No, the New Medicine does not guarantee survival. More importantly though, it allows us to recognize that our lives are "subject" to the 5 Biological Laws of Nature and that we are all going to die one day. We understand health and sickness and that sometimes there is nothing we can do - apart from accepting that we are witnessing the final chapter in someone's life. From a biological point of view, this happens when the extent and/or content of the conflict is just too much or the conflict continues to recur over and over again.

In the big scheme of things, we all know that we are eventually going to die and when someone's time comes, this or any other medicine isn't going to help – this is the just the way fate works.

Unfortunately, there is a double standard: If one single person dies during treatment with the New Medicine, all hell breaks loose: "They would still be alive if they hadn't believed in that nonsense." Not mentioning the cost and despite the countless deaths as a result of conventional medical treatment, their final words are always: "We did our best, but there was nothing more we could do to save them."

What can I do as someone who is affected?

At the beginning, you need to study the biological connections (Internet, books, lectures, seminars). With this knowledge, try to determine the conflict(s), conflict triggers, belief systems and causal conditioning. This knowledge is half the battle. If the cause of the active or recurring conflict has been found, the task at hand is to adjust your emotional life accordingly and, if possible, to bring about a tangible change in the situation. When it comes to making the necessary changes in your life, there is no patented recipe for success. If you can't seem to manage it on your own, it is helpful to enlist the aid of a therapist. An outsider can often see things more clearly than you can yourself (the forest for the trees).

If you are already in the repair phase and it's not a serious case, "riding it out" is usually sufficient, but not always. Sometimes we also need help from nature or some forms of conventional medicine.

Naturally, it's best when you have "internalized" the 5 Biological Laws of Nature, before you get sick. This keeps the shock of the diagnosis and prognosis from being so dramatic and you'll be able to keep a cool head when it comes to making the important decisions about your therapy.

Nobody is spared by biological conflicts. Life is full of surprises and some of them are very difficult to deal with.

Basically, being easy going is surely the best way to navigate through life. However, during the "critical times," when events call our identity into question, we can't always just take things easy and these are the times when most of our conflicts arise.

Closing words

There is no doubt that the knowledge of the 5 Biological Laws will revolutionize medicine. The only question is: How long will the reigning medical-pharmaceutical-media cartel delay this revolution?

Unfortunately, the discourse regarding the New Medicine lacks objectivity. Also, Dr. Hamer's harsh attacks on conventional medicine didn't do anything to improve the situation. On the contrary, they scared away many people who were actually interested in his insights.

Now it's time to bury the hatchet. Accusations won't bring any of our loved ones back and there are still people who continue to suffer. These victims will surely forgive the medical establishment when this monolith finally admits that they were acting in good faith and didn't know any better.

Many physicians are also looking forward to a new age: a time in which they will once again be able to treat people holistically – their souls, spirits and their bodies – a time in which they won't have to resist the temptations of the pharmaceutical industry.

At this point, I can't conclude without mentioning what may be the most important message of all:

The New Medicine is a wonderful thing – it puts medicine on a solid foundation, so much so, that we can we can finally speak about medicine it as a science. However, we shouldn't lose sight of the most beneficial, yet easily overlooked point amidst all of the conflict analyses, Hamer foci, and the growth and degradation of cells:

Love can heal all wounds.

May we practice the New Medicine with, love, joy, sympathy, gratitude and an affinity to God. May we apply this biological knowledge with our knowledge of the power of the family (biological decoding/Bert Hellinger) and the message of the spiritual teachers and their principles – the essence of all religions.

May we also make a bridge to other therapeutic disciplines. Almost all of them warrant consideration and have something valuable to offer us. Only when we are able to do this will the potential of the New Medicine truly unfold.

Reading

- **ThePsychic Roots of Diseases**

Reference book for therapists and patients with over 500 case studies, categorized by organ with color illustrations.

By Björn Eybl, the author of this booklet. xxx pages, XXXX Verlag 2017, ISBN XXXXXXXXXXXXXX.

Available.

- Scientific Chart of Germanic New Medicine® by Dr. Med. Mag. Theol. Ryke Geer Hamer, published by Amici di Dirk, 2006, ISBN 978-84-96127-29-6

- Summary of the German New Medicine by Dr. Med. Ryke Geer Hamer, published by Amici di Dirk, 2000, ISBN 84-930091-9-9
- The Ultimate Conspiracy Theory – The Biomedical Paradigm by James McCumsikey

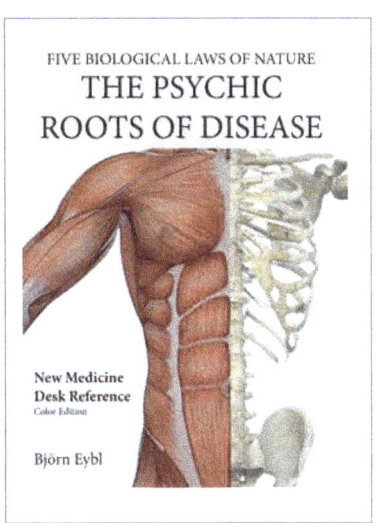

The content and recommendations in this booklet are based on the scientific findings of Dr. Hamer. They are meant for the reader's personal edification; they cannot, however, substitute for the diagnosis and therapy of a competent therapist.

Information on the internet
www.youtube.com/watch?v=3zYWtzq4XBk
(New Medicine and the five biological laws, youtube)
http://www.newmedicine.ca
http://learninggnm.com/
http://www.german-new-medicine-healer.com

Author responsible for the content of this booklet: Bjorn Eybl, Au bei der Traun 53, A-4623 Gunskirchen, Austria.

Translated by Niamh Prior and Andrew Schlademan - many thanks!

For over thirty years we've all been dreaming....
"The New Medicine will break through when the crocuses bloom"

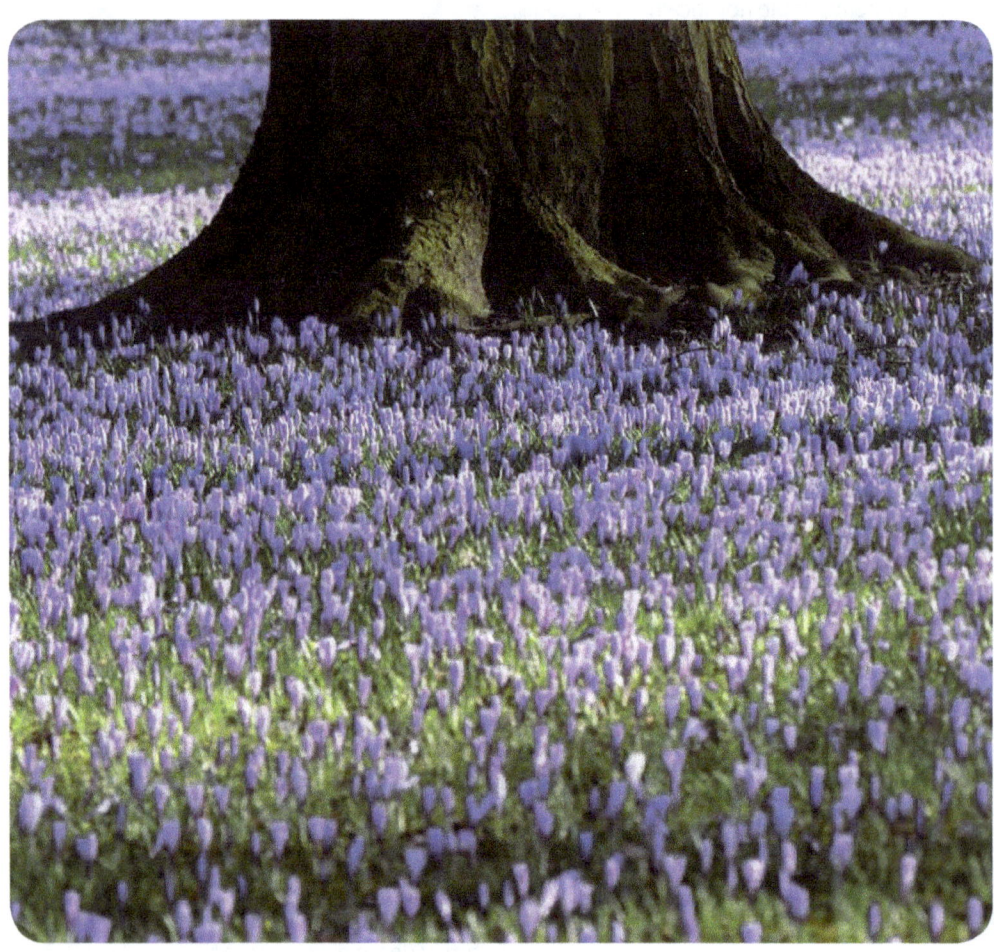

For more information contact

www.ingramcontent.com/pod-product-compliance
Lightning Source LLC
Chambersburg PA
CBHW071729020426
42333CB00017B/2453